I0441597

Anti-Inflammatory Diet

The Ultimate Beginners Guide to Eliminate Body Pain and Restore Your Overall Health By Eating Foods Designed For You

Table of Contents

☐ **Copyright 2016 by Lee Douglas - All rights reserved.**

This document is geared toward providing exact and reliable information in regard to the topic and issue covered. The publication is sold with the idea that the publisher is not required to render accounting, officially permitted, or otherwise, qualified services. If advice is necessary, legal or professional, a practiced individual in the profession should be ordered.

- From a Declaration of Principles that was accepted and approved equally by a Committee of the American Bar Association and a Committee of Publishers and Associations.

In no way is it legal to reproduce, duplicate, or transmit any part of this document in either electronic means or in printed format. Recording of this publication is strictly prohibited and any storage of this document is not allowed unless with written permission from the publisher. All rights reserved.

The information provided herein is stated to be truthful and consistent, in that any liability, in terms of inattention or otherwise, by any usage or abuse of any policies, processes, or directions contained within is the solitary and utter responsibility of the recipient reader. Under no circumstances will any legal responsibility or blame be held against the publisher for any reparation, damages, or monetary loss as a result of the information herein, either directly or indirectly.

Introduction

The stressful lifestyle of the modern today not only robs us of our chance of living a happy and fulfilled life, but it also makes us take a poor care of ourselves and leave the door open for the diseases to swoop in. Have you ever wondered about why the majority of us are so out of condition? Neglecting our needs as human beings results with nothing more, but our own defeat.

How many times have you said to yourself "I am sure it is fine" when you faced some health-concerning issue? Can you really be sure that that sharp pain you just felt is nothing but a false alarm? Of course you can't. Then, what should you do? Should you just accept the fact that your busy daily schedules have made you a bundle of nerves, and go on popping pills just to ease the pain and carry on with your activities? Well, yes, if you aim for a life shorter by many years. But since many of us dream of a healthy retirement let me just stop you right there and ask you one thing "What are you waiting for?". It is time to seek guidance and pull your health problems by the root – the inflammation.

And since every condition is mainly treated with an ANTIdote (see how I've put an accent on this powerful prefix), the only way you can eradicate inflammation is by welcoming an ANTI-inflammatory diet. Still not convinced? Well, go on and read this book to see what an untreated inflammation can result in, why you should choose the anti-inflammatory diet, what you should eat and what belongs in the trash can, and many more reasons that will finally open your eyes.

After all, you know how they say 'an ounce of prevention is worth the pound of cure'.

Inflammation Under the Spotlight

Let's just make something clear from the very start – inflammation is not the same as an infection. Many people think these two are the same when in fact they are two very different health condition. Although infection may be a common cause of inflammation, these processes have nothing in common. Think of the infection as the attacker and inflammation as the defender. The infection is a harmful process that is caused by a virus, fungus or a bacteria that spreads throughout our bodies in the most irritating way. When the body detects the 'attacker', it is trying to create a 'shield' in order to defend itself from harm. This process of the body attempting to protect us from the dangerous stimuli and keep the cells as undamaged as possible is called inflammation.

So why is inflammation bad, some of you may think, when in fact it is a mechanism of defense that keeps us healthy? It is true, in certain situations inflammation can be quite beneficial, actually. When you catch a cold, your body is getting rid of the invaders in the form of a fever – and that is the inflammation. When a mosquito bites you, it itches you, until the inflammation does its work and eliminate the harmful agents. This is called *acute inflammation*. Acute inflammation is known to cause a discomfort (which usually doesn't last longer than a couple of days) until your body eradicates the 'attackers' and makes sure that your health is not affected in a more serious way. But the one we should all watch out for, the inflammation that causes us a great deal of long-term aches and constant pain, is called *chronic inflammation*.

So what exactly is the difference between these two types of inflammation? While the acute inflammation is considered to be good, as it can get rid of the cause, the chronic type is basically the opposite. It occurs when the body fails to eliminate the pathogens guilty for the inflammations and cannot start the process of body healing. Chronic inflammation is when things go wrong. What was supposed to be helpful, now is the reason you are in pain. To bring this explanation closer, think of the chronic type as a flooded apartment. Let's say you dream of relaxing and taking a warm and soothing bath. You leave the water running to fill the tub. A friend calls to tell you there is an emergency. The conversation you just had, occupies your mind completely. You leave the apartment immediately and forget all about the bathtub. Hours later, you come back home only to find your apartment flooded and your wooden floor ruined. You see, what was meant to be good for you, now has caused you a serious problem. The same is with chronic inflammation. After an injury, your body does the best to help you heal, but it often happens that it ends up doing you more harm than good.

What Causes It?

Like I said, it is believed that one of the major causes of inflammation is an infection. And while your doctor may prescribe you some antibiotics to eradicate the bacteria that has infected your bloodstream, that might not be the solution. Of course, it will get rid of the temporary condition, but it will not solve the problem. When inflammation happens, people usually blame it on the virus that has infected them, when in fact, they are the ones to blame for not paying close attention to their bodily changes and not taking a proper health care of themselves.

Even though the bacteria or fungi are the cause of inflammation, they are not what triggers it. Do you know that we have plenty of bacteria living inside our bodies? Some of them are good and help our body to break down some not so useful substances. But some of our the bacteria in our gastrointestinal tract can be our number one enemies. There is a condition that's called *disbyosis* which is basically an imbalance of our gut bacteria that is commonly the reason why inflammation occurs. But your immune system doesn't have to be overreacting to the fungi for them to cause inflammation, and neither you have to be super sensitive to allergies. It is enough to have an improperly balanced diet, lead a reckless lifestyle or to be constantly stressed, to let the inflammation take over your body and 'pollute' your health. Another factor that may, unfortunately, be the cause of inflammation are the toxins that are all around us, whether in the water we drink, the air we breathe or the food we consume.

Because obesity is also commonly associated with inflammation, I want to make something very clear. I have come across people saying how the number that the scale shows is to blame. Obesity as an excess weight condition does not cause inflammation. The condition itself is not a problem. What seems to be the issue with obese people is their poor diet. Unbalanced diet creates too much fat in the body, and carrying that 'damage' is what opens the door to inflammation.

Although inflammation mainly occurs as a self-protective process of the body to fight off the invaders, that is not always how it happens. There are some conditions when inflammation occurs without having irritants to get rid of. In certain situations, the body attacks healthy tissues mistaking them for dangerous intruders and hurtful pathogens. This happens with autoimmune diseases like arthritis, fibromyalgia, psoriasis, type 1 diabetes, lupus, celiac disease, etc.

How to Recognize It?

When there is a group of tiny little germs with pointy spears inside us, our body has no other job, then to do its best to defend us from the potential danger. That is when white blood cells are being released into the bloodstream to prevent the outside attackers from doing us harm. When this mechanism occurs, our body releases an increased amount of bloodstream to the infected or injured part. This results in *redness.* Redness is the most common symptom of inflammation, and it is often accompanied with *warmth.* Usually the released chemicals release fluids, which makes the injured part noticeably *swollen.* So, if some part of your body is red, swollen and somewhat warmer, then you are dealing with inflammation. That means that your body is not only eradicating the irritants, but it is also getting rid of the tissue that the 'attackers' have damaged. Without this kind of inflammation, your wounds will never have the chance to heal properly.

But how to recognize the silent and hazardous inflammation that has not that notable signs and symptoms? There are a few symptoms that are associated with chronic inflammation, but are not that relevant indicator:

- Chronic pain

- Wrinkles and other aging signs

- High blood pressure

- Skin conditions

- Ulcers

- Fatigue

- Asthma

- Allergies

- Red eyes

Even if you have a couple of these symptoms you may not have chronic inflammation, and also, some people may have none of these, but have one. Chronic inflammation is a silent condition that is eating your body alive from the inside, without you being aware of it. Sometimes there are absolutely no signs of inflammation, but that doesn't have to mean you don't have one. It is a kind of a strange process; in certain situations inflammations shows no symptoms and gives you absolutely no heads up before it hits you with a serious disease.

However, if you want to be sure, you can test yourself and see whether there is something strange going on inside your body. Although there isn't a single test that will clearly show whether your health is under attack or not, there are a series of checkups that can offer a pretty solid picture about the way your cells work:

- Test your C-reactive protein. The most reliable marker is the CPR test. A single blood test can sometimes prevent you from a great deal of troubles.

- X-ray results. Sometimes the pain in the joints is due to inflammation. You better check to be sure.

- Check our HDL. Sometimes raised cholesterol occurs due to inflammation.

- Blood sugar test.

- Check the SED rate. The sedimentation rate in the blood sometimes means that there is an inflammatory activity going on.

Health Concerning Risks

Remember how I said that inflammation is at the root of nearly all diseases? Do you have an idea why is that? It is pretty simple actually. Unlike the acute inflammation that helps our wounds and injuries heal, the chronic, low-grade inflammation stays inside our body, and it constantly tries to get rid of the harm. When your immune system is faced with a regular response to inflammation, it will start to wear off, age quickly, and become extremely vulnerable. That makes your body and overall health very susceptible to diseases. Think of an old pair of jeans and compare it to the one you've just bought. All those years of wearing a single piece of clothing resulted in degrading. The same happens in your body. All that 'action' going on inside of you will eventually result in you getting ill.

Inflammation can easily affect all of your internal organs. It is at the core of many diseases, but it is mainly linked to:

- Cancer. A Harvard study performed on teenagers has shown that those with a high rank of inflammation had 63% more chance of developing cancer.

- Heart disease. The white blood cells that are increased during the inflammation's work of 'defeating' the body are attracted to the fatty plaques which will eventually create clots in the blood and will most likely result in heart disease and might eventually cause a heart attack.

- Lung damages. When your lungs are inflamed, even breathing is a hard task to perform. It usually results in chronic pulmonary diseases or asthma.

- Trouble losing weight. Inflammation can slow the metabolism and send false hunger signs and make you gain pounds.

- Diabetes. It is known that inflammation can increase the levels of insulin resistance, which can result in developing diabetes.

- Quick cell aging.

- Depression.

- Bone damages.

- Kidney problems.

- Sleep deprivation.

What About Food?

Unhealthy diet is always to blame. Whether we are talking about not being able to fit into that expensive shirt anymore or have high cholesterol levels, the point is, what we consume mainly dictates what kind of life we will be living. Unfortunately, people usually wait until it's too late to start paying attention to what kind of food will be served on their dinner table. After all, it is impossible to bring back all those years of throwing away broccoli when no one was looking.

Just as with any other health condition, the greatest culprit for developing inflammation is, of course, the poor diet. But, when I say poor diet, I don't only refer to the diet that lacks the necessary nutrients. Quite the contrary actually. I am talking about those 'balanced' diets that cover our nutritional needs, but are also packed with those sweet, addictive dangers that we cannot seem to live without, that are razing everything we are trying to achieve by 'counting calories' and 'eating the rainbows'.

Planning our daily meals carefully is nothing but a waste of time, if we add a few 'forbidden' items here and there. There are types of food that actually cause and worsen inflammation. In order to keep your health from deteriorating, pay attention to the following list of foods that should be off-limits, to keep those cells rejuvenated.

The Top 12 Triggers

To keep inflammation further from your cells, as well as to prevent yourself from developing other chronic diseases, make sure never to include these 12 types of food in your diet:

#1: Sugar. Yes, at the top of every list of foods to ignore is, of course, sugar. So why do we keep skipping this rule? Are we that addicted to adding extra sweetness to our food? Do you really think that our bodies are designed to break down all of that additional sugar we consume? No, they are not. Although it will be hard to resist the temptation of enjoying a creamy piece of cake or drinking a fruit juice, try to skip every product that has 'ose' written on the label (like fructose).

#2: Trans Fats. Do you know that the trans fats can seriously damage our cells and contribute to inflammation? Never buy those products that contain unnatural trans fats because they are hard for the body to process. Stay away from the fries, pizza, donuts, burgers, and cupcakes. And those crackers, too.

#3: MSG. Researches show that Monosodium Glutamate can induce inflammation. Although it is still unknown how it can cause inflammation, experts say that MSG is not something your body can process with ease. That being said, they advise staying away from products containing this additive such as soy sauce. This chemical mostly found in the Asian cuisine is also extremely bad for the liver.

#4: Meat. Don't get me wrong, I am not saying to go vegetarian, I just mean to pay attention to what kind of meat you eat. Avoid the commercially produced you buy at the supermarkets, avoid red meat and processed meat. Also, try not to make the meat the star of the meal. Eat only small portions that you will combine wisely with other healthy foods. Forget poultry from the market, avoid pork, beef, sausages, salami, ham and bacon.

#5: Alcohol. Should I really say something more? I think it is quite obvious what this beverage does to our health. It not only loads the liver, but it also causes inflammation and irritates the larynx. Try to stay away from alcohol completely, but if you feel like having a glass of wine at your friend's wedding, make sure not to ask for a refill.

#6: Milk. Are you aware of the fact that over 60% of the population are lactose intolerant? That is not without a reason. The fact that you may not experience diarrhea and gases does not mean that drinking milk is particularly good for your health. Put its nutrients on the side and focus on what it can cause. Milk is considered to be one of the most common allergens and it can easily induce inflammation.

#7: Omega-6 Fatty Acids. On average, people consume more omega-6 than omega-3 fatty acids. This will only create an imbalance that can contribute to developing inflammation. Forget your usual cooking oils like sunflower, sesame, canola, grape seed or corn oil. Margarine should also not be a part of your diet.

#8: Synthetic Sweeteners. You may think you have done a great job substituting sugar with a synthetic sweetener, when in fact, you may have done nothing more than consuming even more harmful substitutes. Synthetic sweeteners are considered to be guilty of developing many diseases, so stay off Amino sweet, aspartame, saccharin, etc.

#9: Gluten. Gluten is often associated with digestion problems, so in order to avoid that bloating to be the cause of your inflammation, you better join the popularity that has excluded gluten from their diets. Say no to wheat, barley and rye.

#10: Iodized Salt. Although you may not connect sodium with salt at first, this ingredient is actually a part of the salt on your table. Sodium is known to cause kidney problems, but what happens when it stays in the bloodstream just to be accumulated? It actually can be a cause for many inflammatory conditions.

#11: Seasoning Mix. We all love the flavor that a seasoning mix can add to our dishes, but are you aware what these mixes are made of? Do you know they contain a good portion of sugar, as well as artificial coloring? These chemicals can easily induce inflammation. Make your own mixes with some healthy spices instead, to bring out the deliciousness.

#12: Peanuts. Next to milk and gluten, peanuts are also on the list of the world's greatest allergens. It is not rare, for peanuts to be accompanied by fungus, so there is absolutely no need for you to include them in your diet and expose yourself to the risk of developing inflammation for no reason.

Common Mistakes

Even when you think you are consuming a super healthy diet, you might be doing a couple of common mistakes that rob you from getting the most out of the food you eat, and actually contribute to developing inflammation and make you age quicker.

Peeling Your Fruits and Vegetables. Do I really need to go on? We all know how most of the nutrients are actually found in the peel, so why discard it? And while we are all aware how peeling apples and pears is not something we should be doing, the next time you think about stripping away the skin of these foods, you better reconsider that urge:

Bananas – Yes, it sounds kind of gross eating a banana peel, but if you put it in your juicer, I guarantee that you'll be enjoying a healthier and super yummy juice.

Onions – The skin of the onion may not be edible, but adding it to your stock will load your meal with quercetin which promotes anti-inflammation.

Eggplants – Rich in chlorogenic acid, the eggplant skin is packed with anti-inflammatory properties, so make sure not to peel it.

Pineapples – Pineapple skin may be hard to digest rough, but if you add it in a juicer or sauté it for a couple of minutes, you will be getting the most out of its inflammation-decreasing enzyme – bromelain.

Oranges – No, I don't mean to start eating whole and bitter oranges. But instead of peeling and discarding its peel, try grating it and then sprinkle it on top of your salad. It is packed with anti-inflammatory properties.

Cooking With Olive Oil. Although we said how you should avoid the usual cooking oils, that does not mean that cooking everything with olive oil is healthy for your diet. Although extra virgin olive oil must be a part of your anti-inflammatory diet, it is not always a good idea to cook with it. Never heat olive oil above 250 degrees, as it starts to break down its good fatty acids and it will start to smoke. Drizzle it over fresh food instead.

Falling For the Frozen-Veggies-Are-Bad Myth. What it seems to be the biggest confusion when it comes to eating vegetables, is that you should avoid frozen veggies. Of course, you should always try to eat as fresh as possible, but sometimes the frozen ones are healthier than the fresh ones from the supermarket. You see, frozen vegetables are picked at their prime and frozen, so all of their nutrients are preserved, while those you see in the market, may have been standing there for a few days.

Boiling Vegetables. While boiling may be the fastest way to cook your broccoli, know that by doing that you are leaving most of the vegetable's nutrients in the cooking water. This may be good if you plan on making a soup, but, if you want to discard the water and eat only the vegetables, choose another cooking option like steaming or stir frying.

Using Too Much No-Grain Flour. While coconut and almond flour may be a much healthier substitution for grain flour, if you go crazy with this ingredient, it may result in some not-so-healthy consequences. Almond flour contains omega 6 fatty acids, so if you do not consume it moderately, it will contribute to developing inflammation.

Fight Inflammation Naturally

The number of health gurus that advise the natural approach for fighting inflammation is rising every day. Choosing to go off medications and shift to a more beneficial treatment by taking what nature has to offer, is the only way you will get rid of not only inflammation but many other health conditions as well. To put aside the chemicals that will end up harming you instead of helping you, treating inflammation with medication will not solve the problem, simply because inflammation is usually at the root of many issues that are going on inside of your body. Are you really up for a handful of pills before or after each meal to try to fight off every health problem at once? Or are you simply going to flush those pills down the drain, and change the medical specialist who has failed to find the perfect solution for you?

Inflammation is a very treatable condition, and if approached the right way, it can reward you with a long and peaceful life. So, are you ready to take the matter into your own hands? Read on to see how you can stop those wrinkles from appearing and keep the smile on your face.

The Importance of Anti-Inflammatory Diet

It is easier to go through life eating what is available to you, not paying attention to the problems that those unhealthy choices may be causing you. There is nothing that can compare to satisfying your cravings or not resisting the temptation. But, all of those sweet pleasures come with a price – your life. And since we cannot put a price on our lives, I say we better pull up our sleeves and start fighting for our health.

When feeling that heat from the inflammation, there is absolutely no room for mistakes. From now on, the food you eat will be pulling the strings. So, to make sure that there are only good bacteria left in your gut, it is time to make changes in your diet. But before we go on, let me explain to you what this diet is and what isn't, first.

What anti-inflammatory diet is not:

- Anti-inflammatory diet is not a diet that will help you get into that old pair of jeans in no time. Its goal is not fast shedding pounds, but retrieving health. Although getting rid of the fat-based foods and other unhealthy ingredients will help you eventually lose weight and have a slim body, do not expect instant results.

- It is not a one of a kind diet. There are foods to avoid and foods to include, and you get to make your own meal plans. (In the following chapter you will find menu ideas and recipes that can be the basis of your diet). There are many anti-inflammatory diets, and each of them has its own plan.

- It is not the same as the Mediterranean diet. Although these two diets have many similarities, and anti-inflammatory diet may be mainly based on the ingredients of the Mediterranean diet (fish, vegetables, fruit and olive oil), know that this kind of diet has much more restrictions and also a couple of extras. Plus anti-inflammatory diet is cheaper.

What anti-inflammatory diet is:

- A beneficial diet that will reduce inflammation

- A diet that decreases chronic pain

- Anti-inflammatory diet prolongs the aging process

- It lowers the risk of many diseases

- Keeps your weight in check

- Uplifts your mood

Your New Shopping List

Now that you have learned what you have to do in order to get rid of inflammation, eliminate pain and improve your health in general, it is time to clean your fridge, kitchen and pantry from the potential dangers, and make room for the new stars of your diet.

From now on, when you enter a grocery store there will be some aisles you will avoid, and fill your shopping cart with healthy ingredients only. Let's get you prepared for your next grocery shopping, by creating your new shopping list:

Dark Leafy Greens. Spinach, bok choy, kale and Swiss Chard are known to be rich in antioxidants called flavonoids that can restore the health of your cells and stop inflammation. Dark leafy greens are also packed with vitamin E, which, according to many researches, protects from the molecules called cytokines that promote inflammation.

Tea. Replace your cup of coffee with green or black tea and you are one step closer to getting rid of the inflammation. Also rich in flavonoids and other properties that protect from inflammation, a package of green or black tea must be in your shopping cart.

Extra Virgin Olive Oil. The compound oleocanthal found in extra virgin olive oil has the same effect on inflammation as ibuprofen. This centerpiece of the Meditteranean diet has also many other health improving properties, so if you are a fan of it, please do not hold back. Dunk your pieces of bread into it, drizzle over salads and vegetables for getting its amazing benefits.

Blueberries. Loaded with quercetin, blueberries are one of the top foods that fight inflammation. Studies have shown that quercetin can make significant health improvements in people suffering from inflammation. Make sure to include this antioxidant in your diet.

Beets. Beets have multiple beneficial properties. Packed with the antioxidant called batalin, beets can repair cells and fight inflammation. Another amazing property of the beets is magnesium, and since, the lack of magnesium is linked with many inflammatory conditions, you can be sure that beets will be of great help in your fight with inflammation.

Fatty Fish. Salmon, sardines, mackerel, tuna and other oily fish are the perfect dinner choice when trying to get rid of the inflammation. They are rich in omega-3 fatty acids, which are known to fight inflammation. This powerful component of the fish is really in the heart of the anti-inflammatory diet, so if you do not eat fish, you might want to consider some fish-oil supplements.

Ginger. If you are a fan of this root and add ginger spice in almost every dish, well here are some amazing news for you. Studies have shown that the incredible properties of the ginger root help in the inflammation fighting process, as well as releasing joint pain caused by arthritis. It is not really clear how this ingredient contributes to decreasing inflammations, but many experts believe we should thank its gingerol compound.

Dark Chocolate. If you thought that this diet will rob you from the thing you like most – chocolate, well, think again. One Italian study has shown that eating one square of dark chocolate every day, has more successful results in fighting inflammation than not eating chocolate at all. It is also rich in flavonoids. However beneficial its properties, make sure to be moderate.

Tomatoes. Flashy and juicy tomatoes are known to reduce inflammation, especially in the lungs, thanks to the compound lypocene. A great fact is that tomatoes contain even more lypocene when they are cooked, so bring out the Italian in you and make some delicious tomato sauce. Make tomato juice and drink a glass daily before breakfast.

Turmeric. Besides adding a delightful flavor to our meals, this yellow spice has yet another benefit. It improves our health. Turmeric is known to reduce inflammation, lower pain and reduce the stiffness in arthritis conditions, thanks to its substance called curcumin. As a powerful ally in your battle with inflammation, I suggest you adding this spice to your meals every day.

Onions and Garlic. As I already mentioned how onions contain the antioxidant quercetin, I suggest you to increase your consumption of this beneficial ingredient. Garlic is also known for preventing inflammation to take over.

Broccoli. Being such a healthy and beneficial vegetable, it is no surprise that broccoli should be a part of your grocery shopping list. This ultimate superfood contains many vitamins and antioxidants that also decrease inflammation and prolong aging.

Probiotic Foods. Many times inflammation occurs due to microbial imbalances, so bringing balance back to the gastrointensinal tract, can purge the inflammation out of your gut. Probiotic foods like kefir, sauerkraut and kimchi can help you with this task.

Bone Broth. The broth from boiling beef bones in water for hours is extremely helpful for your health. This beneficial liquid is packed with collagen, which stops your immune systems from working on autopilot and attacking healthy cells. Bone broth is also rich in chondroitin sulfates, it will relieve the joint pain and fights inflammation.

Soy. Studies have shown that thanks to the compounds called isoflavones, soy can lower the CPR levels in women and decrease inflammation. Do not go for products where soy is heavily processed. Choose ingredients like tofu and edamame.

Anti-Inflammatory Diet Plan

I believe that with the content of the previous chapters I have managed to boost your confidence and motivate you to throw those unhealthy snacks in the trash can, and that your fridge is now loaded with fresh ingredients and has all the colors of the rainbow. But this wouldn't be THE ULTIMATE GUIDE if my assistance stopped right there. In this final chapter, I will also provide you with some healthy recipes for breakfast, lunch and dinner that can get you started.

But before you start showing off your cooking skills, let me reveal to you which rules you must follow, while creating your new anti-inflammatory menu:

- Ban processed and refined fruit from your diet.

- Put the emphasis on fresh fruit and vegetables.

- Your anti-inflammatory diet should be based on 2000-3000 calories daily.

- 40% - 50% of your daily intake should be carbs, 30% fat and 20% - 30% daily intake of proteins.

- It is recommended that your diet is free of allergens (aim for as little allergens as possible).

- Eat fish 3 times a week.

- Sweeten your meals the natural way, by adding fruits that are phytonutrient-rich, such as apples, berries, and apricots.

- Flavor your meals with healthy spices; do not use salt.

- Aim for at least 1 ounce of fiber daily.

- All foods rich in omega-3 acids are welcome.

- Eat only home-made meals.

- Drink plenty of pure water.

- Know the products you buy. Read the labels carefully.

- Aim for organic food.

- Choose a local farmer you trust, who will supply you with the freshest ingredients.

Recipes for Fighting Inflammation and Staying Young

To ensure you will get the right anti-inflammatory properties and that you start your journey the proper way, below you will find 21 recipes that will cover each meal for one whole week. During the first week, you will learn the basis of the anti-inflammatory cooking, learn great new recipes, as well as get some experience that will help you get creative and make your own recipes. Feel free to modify the following recipes up to your own personal taste; you can omit or add some ingredients, just be sure to follow the rules of the anti-inflammatory diet.

Besides the fact that they will reduce the inflammation and improve your health, these next 21 recipes will also stop the aging process. Now, grab your apron and start cooking.

Breakfast

The main rule of every diet is – never skip breakfast. The most important meal of the day should energize and pack you with the necessary nutrients that will get you going. Here are some anti-inflammatory breakfast recipes you can try.

Day 1: Gingerbread Apple Oatmeal

Ingredients:
4 cups Water
1 cup Oats, steel cut
1/3 cup grated Apple
¼ tsp ground Ginger
1 ½ tsp ground Cinnamon
1 tsp ground Cloves
1/8 tsp ground Nutmeg
¼ tsp ground Coriander
¼ tsp ground Allspice
¼ tsp ground Cardamom

Preparation:
1. Cook the oats following the package's instruction; add all the spices along with the oats.
2. Remove from heat and let sit for 2 minutes.
3. Stir in the grated apple.
4. Enjoy.

Day 2: Protein Pineapple Smoothie

Ingredients:
1 cup Pineapple chunks, preferably frozen
2 cups Spinach (Kale works just fine, too)

1 cup Green Tea, cooled
½ cup Mango chunks, preferably frozen
2/3 Cucumber, cut into chunks
1/2 Banana, cut into chunks
3 Mint Leaves
½ inch Ginger Root, peeled
1 scoop Protein Powder
¼ tsp ground Turmeric
1 tbsp Chia Seeds
5 ice Cubes

Preparation:
1. Place all of the ingredients, except chia seeds in a blender.
2. Blend until smooth.
3. Add the chia seeds and blend for 2 more seconds, just to combine them well.
4. Add more ice cubes if you like it to be thicker.
5. Enjoy.

Day 3: Berry Crapes

Ingredients:
2 Eggs
½ cup Water
½ cup Nut Milk
1 cup gluten-free Flour
2 tbsp Coconut Oil, plus 1 tbsp for the pan
1 ½ tbsp Agave Nectar

4 tbsp non-fat Plain Yogurt
½ cup Fresh Berries, mashed

Preparation:
1. Place 2 tbsp of coconut oil in a pan.
2. Melt it over medium heat.
3. In a bowl, whisk the eggs, nut milk, water and agave nectar, until well combined.
4. Gradually whisk in the flour.
5. Whisk in the melted coconut oil.
6. In a pan, melt a small amount of the remaining coconut oil, just to ensure the crepe will not stick to the pan.
7. Pour 1/3 of the crepe batter into the pan. Swirl to cover the pan surface.
8. Cook until lightly browned.
9. Flip and cook the other side.
10. Repeat the same process with the remaining batter.
11. Combine the yogurt and mashed berries.
12. Divide the 'sauce' between the crepes.
13. Roll them up.
14. Enjoy.

Day 4: Quinoa Spinach Omelette Bites

Ingredients:
1 cup cooked Quinoa
2 Eggs

1/3 cup chopped Spinach
½ cup crumbled Tofu
1 tbsp chopped Parsley
½ tsp Black Pepper
½ tsp Oregano

Preparation:
1. Preheat your oven to 350 degrees F.
2. Grease your muffin tin with coconut oil.
3. Mix the quinoa, eggs, and tofu in a bowl.
4. Stir in the rest of the ingredients.
5. Fill your muffin tins to the top with the mixture.
6. Bake for about 20 minutes.
7. Remove the bites from the oven and let cool for about 15 minutes.
8. With the help of a small knife, remove them from the tin.
9. Serve and enjoy.

Day 5: Spanish Fritata

Ingredients:
12 Organic Eggs
2 tbsp Coconut Oil
1 cup Spinach

1 Small Red Onion, finely chopped
½ cup Mushrooms
Pinch of Black Pepper
½ tsp Favorite Spice

Preparation:
1. Preheat your oven to 375 degrees F.
2. Melt the coconut oil in a pan over medium heat.
3. Add the onion and sauté for 3 minutes.
4. Stir in the mushrooms and sauté until soft.
5. Add spinach and cook until wilted.
6. Remove the veggies from the pan and set aside.
7. Return the pan to the heat; lower from medium to low heat.
8. Combine the eggs and coconut milk, add the spices and whisk.
9. Add the eggs to the pan.
10. Mix with a spatula to cook them evenly.
11. Top the eggs with the vegetables.
12. Bake for about 5 minutes.
13. Run a knife through the edges.
14. Place a plate over the pan.
15. Invert the fritata.
16. Serve and enjoy.

Day 6: Blueberry Coconut Porridge

Ingredients:
1 ½ cup Oats
Coconut Shavings, to taste

Blueberries, to taste
2 tbsp Dark Chocolate Shavings
4 tbsp Chia Seeds
3 ½ cups Coconut Milk

Preparation:
1. In a saucepan, combine the coconut milk, oats, and chia seeds.
2. Place it over medium heat; bring to a boil.
3. Reduce the heat to low and simmer until cooked.
4. Transfer to a bowl.
5. Top with chocolate, blueberries and coconut shavings.
6. Enjoy.

Day 7: Avocado Egg Toast

Ingredients:
1 slice of Bread, gluten-free
Half an Avocado
1 ½ tsp of Ghee
1 poached Egg
Red Pepper Flakes

Preparation:
1. Toast the bread.
2. Spread ghee over.
3. Slice the avocado.
4. Arrange the slices on the bread.

5. Top with poached egg.

6. Sprinkle with red pepper flakes.

7. Enjoy.

Lunch

Make some of these simple and delightful lunch recipes that will keep you satisfied until dinner:

Day 1: Sweet Potato and Roasted Red Pepper Soup

Ingredients:

2 tbsp Coconut Oil

2 Onions, chopped

1 jar Roasted Red Peppers

3-4 cups cubed Sweet Potatoes

2 tsp ground Cumin

4 cups Homemade Vegetable Broth

2 tbsp minced Cilantro

1 tsp ground Coriander

1 tbsp Lemon Juice

4 ounces Tofu, cubed

1 can Green Chilies, diced

Preparation:

1. In a large pot, heat the coconut oil.

2. Cook the onions until soft.

3. Add the chiles, red peppers, coriander, and cumin,

and cook for 2 minutes.
4. Stir in the vegetable broth and sweet potatoes.
5. Bring to a boil.
6. Lower the heat and cover the pot.
7. Cook for about 15 minutes.
8. Stir in lemon juice and cilantro.
9. Pour half of the soup in a blender along with the tofu.
10. Blend until smooth.
11. Return to the pot and stir to combine.
12. Serve and Enjoy.

Day 2: Squash and Red Lentil Curried Stew

Ingredients:
1 tsp Coconut Oil
3 Garlic Cloves, minced
1 Onion, chopped
1 cup Red Lentils
4 cups Homemade Vegetable Broth
3 cups cooked Squash
1 cup Dark Leafy Greens
1 tbsp Curry Powder
Pinch of Ginger Powder
½ tsp Black Pepper

Preparation:
1. Heat the coconut oil in a large pot.
2. Saute the onion and garlic for about 5 minutes.

3. Stir in curry powder and cook for an additional minute.
4. Pour the broth and add the lentils.
6. Bring to a boil; reduce the heat and cover.
7. Stir in greens and squash.
8. Cook for 6-7 minutes.
9. Season with pepper and ginger.
10. Serve and enjoy.

Day 3: Avocado and Tuna Salad

Ingredients:
1 can Tuna, in water
¼ Red Onion, chopped
1 Celery Stalk, chopped
1 small Avocado, chopped
Juice of half a Lemon
Pinch of Black Pepper
Extra Virgin Olive Oil, to taste

Preparation:
1. Combine all of the ingredients in a salad bowl.
2. Drizzle EVOO over.
3. Enjoy.

Day 4: Kale Chicken Wraps

Ingredients:
6 cups Kale, chopped
8 ounces Grilled Chicken
1 cup quartered Cherry Tomatoes
1 Garlic Clove, minced
1/8 cup Lemon Juice
1/8 cup Extra Virgin Olive Oil
½ tsp Dijon Mustard
2 Tortillas, gluten-free
Black Pepper, to taste
Red Pepper Flakes, to taste

Preparation:
1. Mix the olive oil, lemon juice, mustard, and garlic.
2. Season with black pepper and red pepper flakes.
3. Add the chicken, kale and cherry tomatoes.
4. Stir to combine.
5. Spread the mixture over the tortillas.
6. Wrap them up and slice in half.
7. Serve and enjoy.

Day 5: Fruit Salad

Ingredients:
2 Pears, cut in cubes
½ cup Grapes
½ cup Pecans
2 Plums, cut into chunks
1/2 Apple, cut in cubes
½ cup chopped Figs

2 tbsp Agave Nectar
1 tbsp Pomegranate Vinegar
1 tbsp Coconut Oil

Preparation:
1. Combine the agave nectar, coconut oil and vinegar in a salad bowl.
2. Toss fruit with the dressing in the bowl.
3 Top with pecans.
4. Enjoy.

Day 6: Roasted Root Vegetables

Ingredients:
2 pounds Roots (Beets, Sweet Potatoes, Parsnips, Carrots)
1 Onion, cut into wedges
3 Garlic Cloves
Chopped herbs (Rosemary, Thyme, Basil)
1 tbsp Extra Virgin Olive Oil
Spices, to taste

Preparation:
1. Preheat your oven to 400 degrees F.
2. Place the roots and onion in a roasting pan.
3. Drizzle oil over.
4. Roast for 45 minutes total; stir after every 15.
5. 15 minutes before the end, add the garlic cloves.
6. 5 minutes before the end, add the herbs.
7. Serve and enjoy.

Day 7: Eggplant – Walnut Pate

Ingredients:
1 Large Eggplant
1 cup Walnuts
2 mashed Garlic Cloves
2 tsp grated Ginger
1/8 tsp Allspice
1 tbsp Extra Virgin Olive Oil
Black Pepper, to taste
Toasted Gluten-Free Bread

Preparation:
1. Preheat the oven to 450 degrees F.
2. Pierce the eggplant with a fork a couple of times.
3. Bake for about 45 minutes.
4. Place the walnuts in a processor and process until finely ground.
5. Remove the eggplant from the oven.
6. Let cool for a little bit.
7. Scrape the flesh into the processor.
8. Add the remaining ingredients.
9. Transfer to a serving bowl.
10. Chill for a couple of hours.
11. Serve with toasted bread for a quick lunch.
12. Enjoy.

Dinner

The richest meal of the day and the one that is worth waiting for is, of course, dinner. If you thought that anti-inflammatory diet will keep you away from enjoying irresistible delicacies, then think again. These next 7 recipes will show you that this healthy diet can indeed provide you with delicious meals that are bursting with flavor:

Day 1: Seared Salmon with Orange Glaze

Ingredients:
6 Salmon Fillets
¼ cup White Wine
3 tbsp Sherry
2 slices of Orange
1 tbsp Sesame Oil
1 cup Fresh Orange Juice
1 tsp Orange Zest
½ tsp grated Ginger

Preparation:
1. Sear the salmon in a skillet with sesame oil for about one minute on each side.
2. Remove them from the skillet; set aside in a baking dish.
3. Drizzle the white wine over the salmon.
4. Bake for about 10 minutes in a previously preheated oven to 400 degrees F.
5. In a saucepan over medium heat, heat the orange juice, ginger, zest and sherry.
6. When the liquid is reduced by half, add the

orange slices and stir.

7. Pour the orange sauce over the salmon.

8. Serve and enjoy.

Day 2: Broccoli Pasta

Ingredients:

1 pound Broccoli

¼ cup Extra Virgin Olive Oil

1 pound gluten-free Pasta

2 tbsp Capers plus 1 tbsp of the Brine

5 Garlic Cloves, minced

1 tsp Red Pepper Flakes

1 cup Parmesan Cheese

Chopped Parsley

Preparation:

1. Trim the ends and cut the broccoli into chunks.

2. Heat the oil in a skillet over medium heat.

3. Add garlic and red pepper flakes and cook no longer than a minute, until fragrant (make sure not to overheat the olive oil.)

4. Add the pasta in a pot with boiling water and cook according to the package instructions. Before the end, add the broccoli and cook until tender. (Be careful, your pasta should be al dente.)

5. Drain the pasta and broccoli.

6. Add capers, brine and ¾ cup Parmesan.

7. Serve topped with the remaining Parmesan

cheese.
8. Sprinkle with chopped parsley.
9. Enjoy.

Day 3: Scallion Black Rice with Peas

Ingredients:
3 cups cooked Black Rice
2 tbsp Coconut Oil
1 bunch Scallions, sliced, whites and greens
separated
1 Yellow Onion, diced
2 Carrots, diced
2 Garlic Cloves, minced
1 tbsp minced Ginger
2 Eggs, beaten
2 tsp toasted Sesame Oil
1 cup sliced Snap Peas
1 tsp Srirarcha
1 tbsp Organic Shelled Hemp Seed
3 tbsp Liquid Aminos

Preparation:
1. Heat the coconut oil in a wok.
2. Saute the carrots, onion and white scallions for
about 5 minutes.
3. Add garlic, snap peas, green scallions, and
ginger, and cook for about 2 minutes.
4. Fold in the rice.

5. After 3 minutes, add the liquid aminos, srirarcha, and sesame oil.
6. Make a well in the center and pour the eggs in.
7. Cook while stirring constantly.
8. Serve and enjoy.

Day 4:Baked Tilapia with Pecan Topping

Ingredients:
4 Tilapia Fillets
1/3 cup chopped Pecans
2 tsp Rosemary, chopped
1/3 cup gluten-free Breadcrumbs
1 Egg White, whisked
1 ½ tsp Extra Virgin Olive Oil
A pinch of cayenne Pepper

Preparation:
1. Preheat your oven to 375 degrees F.
2. In a small dish, combine the bread crumbs, cayenne pepper, olive oil, and pecans.
3. Place the pecan mixture in the oven and bake until golden, about 7 minutes.
4. Dip each fillet in egg white and then into the pecan mixture; arrange them on a greased baking dish.
5. Bake for about 10 minutes.
6. Sprinkle with rosemary.
7. Serve and enjoy.

Day 5: Turkey and Quinoa Bell Peppers

Ingredients:
3 Yellow Peppers
1 pound lean Ground Turkey
1 cup diced Mushrooms
1 cup Tomato Sauce
1 cup cooked Quinoa
1 cup Fresh Spinach
¼ cup diced Onion
2 tsp minced Garlic
1 cup Water
1 ½ tbsp Coconut Oil

Preparation:
1. Saute the vegetables in coconut oil in a pan over medium heat.
2. After 4 minutes, add turkey and garlic.
3. When cooked through, add tomato sauce and ½ cup water.
4. Preheat your oven to 400 degrees F.
5. Fold the quinoa in the pan.
6. Cut the peppers in half.
7. Stuff each half with the turkey and quinoa mixture.
8. Arrange them on a baking dish.
9. Pour the remaining water into the dish.
10. Cover the dish with foil and bake for about half

an hour.

11.Serve and enjoy.

Day 6: Spicy Potatoes and Chicken with Turmeric and Cumin

Ingredients:
1 ½ pounds Yukon Gold Potatoes
1/8 tsp Asafetida
5 tbsp Coconut Oil
½ tsp Mustard Seeds
¼ tsp Chili Powder
½ tsp ground Coriander Seeds
½ tsp Ground Turmeric
½ tsp whole Cumin seeds
3 cups cooked shredded Chicken

Preparation:
1. Cut the potatoes into chunks.
2. Heat the coconut oil in a skillet over medium heat.
3. Add asafetida, then mustard seeds, then cumin.
4. Add the potatoes and stir to combine.
5. Sprinkle turmeric.
6. Cook for about 15 minutes, until cooked.
7. Stir in the chicken and turmeric and cook for 3 more minutes.
8. Serve and enjoy.

Day 7: Mediterranean Salmon Skewers

Ingredients:
½ cup Extra Virgin Olive Oil
¾ pound Salmon, cut into cubes
1 Garlic Clove, minced
1 tbsp chopped Fresh Mint
1 tsp Lime Zest
1 tbsp Lime Juice
2 tbsp chopped Oregano
12 Cremini Mushrooms, quartered
1 cup Broccoli Florets
½ cup Kalamata Olives,
8 wooden skewers, soaked in water

Preparation:
1. Preheat your oven to 375 degrees.
2. Combine the oil, garlic, mint, oregano, lime juice and zest, in a small bowl.
3. Place the salmon, mushrooms, and broccoli in a baking dish.
4. Pour the marinade over and stir to combine.
5. Layer the salmon, mushrooms, broccoli and olive on the skewers.
6. Bake for about 25 minutes in the baking pan.
7. Enjoy.

Conclusion

With a couple of simple changes in your diet, you can move towards a much healthier life where you will not only be relieved from the pain and soreness that inflammation causes, but you will also go through life with the smallest possible risk of developing a life-threatening disease. And to know that you can dodge such hazards, today, it is a rare gift.

So please, cherish the knowledge you have, implement this new anti-inflammatory diet, and use it to live a long and fulfilling life.

Rest assured that you will get to live your old days hale and hearty.

Free Bonus

As Promised Here Is Your Guide To Managing Stress: Discover The Simple Solutions to Live A Stress Free Life.

CLICK HERE to get Your Copy

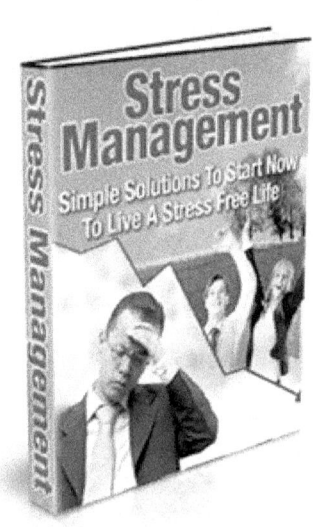

LEARN HOW TO MANAGE YOUR STRESS

Stress can take a huge chunk of your time, energy, and health. Not only your personal relationships suffer, but so as your career and total wellness. Are you struggling from stress? This book explains the true definition of stress, the symptoms and the right way to cure it. Moreover, the book gives tactical strategies to decrease your stress and increase living a happier and healthier life.

Download "Stress Management" For FREE

If You Want Free Best Selling Kindle Books Delivered Straight To Your Inbox

JOIN OUR FREE KINDLE BOOK CLUB!

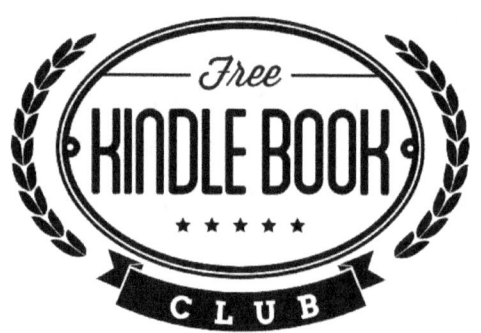

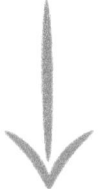

CLICK HERE

BEFORE YOU GO

If you liked this book you may like these other books from Lee Douglas

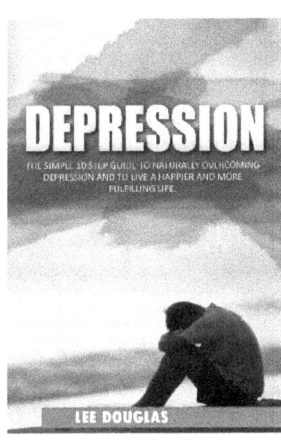

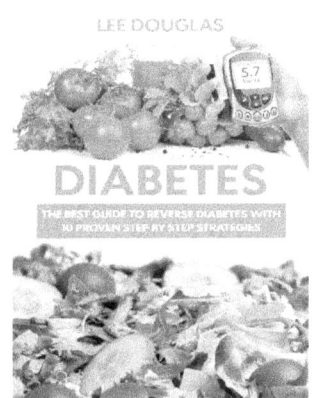

Check out more books by Lee Douglas

BOOKS BY LEE DOUGLAS

Knowledge is Power

Many studies have shown that most people diagnosed with diabetes are actually ignorant about what is really happening in their bodies. It seems pretty impossible to fight off a disease if you are not fully aware of it, don't you think?

People don't say that knowledge is power for no reason. In this case, knowledge about this horrible life-threatening disease will give you the power to make permanent positive changes. Knowing what you're dealing with will make you accept these next steps more willingly in order to reverse or dodge diabetes.

What is diabetes? Unfortunately, diabetes is a chronic life-long condition where your body is incapable of using the amount of glucose properly, so it keeps piling up in your blood. How and why does it happen? To make it clearer, imagine fuel. Yes, fuel. Just like your car needs fuel to get from A to B, the same way your body needs fuel to perform every task, whether it's sleeping or running a marathon. Our body gets most of the fuel from the *glucose*. Once the food we've eaten is converted into glucose, it travels into our body (especially the liver and muscles) and brain, through our bloodstream. Glucose cannot enter our body cells without the hormone *insulin* that the pancreas produces. So when diabetes occurs and glucose is loaded in our blood, is due to the pancreas' inability to produce enough or any insulin.

There are two types of diabetes:

Type 1 Diabetes is a disease where the immune system attacks the healthy beta cells from the pancreas that produce insulin because they are mistaken for bad invaders. This autoimmune condition causes damage to the pancreas that leads to cells' inability to create the required or in some cases any amount of insulin. This type is also called *juvenile* diabetes because it mostly attacks young adults and children. It accounts for 5-10 % of the people diagnosed with diabetes. Although it is hard to reverse, the steps that this guide provide will help people with type 1 diabetes regulate their 'blood sugar' and feel much better overall.

Type 2 Diabetes is a condition where the cells are resistant to insulin. The body keeps up for some time by creating more than enough insulin, which will eventually lead to burned out receptors' sites. Because the cells do not accept the insulin any longer, the glucose cannot be transferred to the brain and body parts, and stays in the bloodstream. This is why the 'blood glucose' or as we call it 'blood sugar' levels are high. Type 2 occurs in 90% of the cases.

There are many people who are under attack by this disease, but are unaware that are diabetic.

How to tell if you show signs of having diabetes? These are the most common symptoms that should ring an alarm that it's time for a medical checkup:

- Frequent urination

- Increased thirst

- Fatigue

- Unexplained weight loss

- Blurry vision

- Poor wound healing

- Extreme hunger

- Irritability

- Tingling in your feet and/or hands

For those of you who aren't diagnosed with diabetes and are reading this guide solely for educational purposes or are in pursuit of advice for someone close to you that is suffering from diabetes - it is critical that you also test yourself and determine whether you are really not confronting diabetes. It is crucial to do so, especially if you are affected by some of the diabetes' <u>risk factors</u>:

- You are overweight

- Have a close family member with diabetes

- Your HDL cholesterol is lower than 35 and your triglycerides level higher than 245

- Your blood pressure is higher than 140/90

- You are older than 45

- Your family background is African American, Hispanic American/Latino, Pacific Islander, Asian American or American Indian

- You had gestational diabetes during pregnancy

- Gave birth to a baby weighing more than 9 pounds

- You are physically inactive

However, even when you decide to test yourself, you should know exactly how to do it. Most doctors have been trained that when a patient wants to be tested for diabetes, they simply measure the glucose levels in their blood, 8 hours after their last meal. Do not get me wrong, this is a relevant test that clearly shows if someone has diabetes, it is just a poor indicator. Diabetes starts long before the *fasting glucose plasma test* confirms so. Now that we have explained how this horrible disease is created, you can only guess that the key to what has gone haywire is, in fact, the insulin. So, instead of measuring the 'sugar' in your blood, which is clearly not at the root of what has gone wrong, ask your doctor for an *insulin response test*. Do not wait for your doctor to diagnose you with diabetes and put you on medication if you have the chance to

eradicate the process. If this test's results show high insulin, you WILL HAVE a chance to normalize it by following our next steps and stop diabetes from occurring.

Be Nutrition-Smart

It is scary. Receiving the news that you are affected by diabetes must definitely be one of the worst moments in your life. You know that it cannot be treated, and you're labeled as diabetic for life. You have seen people struggle with this disease before and you must feel like the end of the world is coming. But it's not.

Although diabetes was known as irreversible for a long time, science has proven otherwise. You CAN reprogram your body so it can begin regulating the blood sugar again. Attacking this disease on the front of food consumption armed with properly balanced diet, you will force your body to repair the damage that diabetes has caused and make the glucose return to normal range, which will lead to its complete reversion. Your nutrition plays a major, if not the most important part when trying to fight off diabetes.

Resist the Temptation

Learning how to say NO to the juicy and delicious, but extremely unhealthy junk food is crucial for reversing diabetes. It's about time to fill your trash can with the fat-bombs lying around your house. You will also have to say goodbye to:

Sugar. When struggling with a blood sugar disease it is pretty clear that sugar is off limits. And when I say sugar, I do not mean just skipping the teaspoon in your tea or coffee cup; I also mean avoiding anything that contains refined sugar. Thinking about substituting it with raw honey? You might want to rethink this urge. Although honey or maple syrup might be slightly healthier versions - they still badly affect the glucose in your blood. Switch to stevia and say farewell to sweet food and beverages.

Grains. Wheat and other grains that contain gluten should be avoided at all times. They are packed with a huge amount of carbohydrates which can easily be broken into sugar only after a couple of minutes after they've been consumed. The intestinal inflammation that gluten causes lead to glucose's spikes.

Conventional Cow's Milk. Dairy is amazing at balancing the sugar in your blood, but not if it comes from conventional cows. This is especially important for those who suffer from type 1 diabetes. The milk from conventional cows harms the body the same way that gluten does. Substitute it with sheep's or goat's milk and enjoy your favorite drink. Always purchase organic and raw milk.

Processed Food. Food loses most of its nutrients in the process of cooking, which can easily lead to inflammation, liver toxification and of course high levels of blood sugar. That being said, you should avoid processed and go for whole foods that will help you reverse diabetes.

You should also exclude dry fruit, soy, canola, packaged food, pretzels, butter and all kinds of frozen pre-cooked food from your diet.

Balance Your Diet

'What to eat now?' Besides the obvious 'why me' question, this must be the first thing that pops up into your mind on your way home from the doctor's office where you've been told the bad news. Living with this disease and being careful about the food you consume, doesn't need to make you feel deprived. Taking a healthy approach and making smart choices about nutrition doesn't have to be exhaustive. If you think that balancing your diet means eating boring and tasteless meals, you are so wrong. Once you get the hang of consuming healthy and properly balanced food, you can dig in to a variety of delightful dishes.

Make these superfoods your ultimate weapon in the kitchen and enjoy a challenging cooking that will reward you with reversed diabetes and improved overall health:

Green Vegetables are the most important food to focus on in order to reverse diabetes. Nutrient- dense, cruciferous, leafy greens and other green vegetables contribute to lower HbA1c (glycated hemoglobin) levels.

Non-Starchy Vegetables like eggplants, mushrooms, onions, peppers, garlic, etc. are packed with phytochemicals and fiber and have effects on blood sugar that are almost nonexistent.

Nuts are a very beneficial superfood to diabetes, as well as our general health. Besides the fact that they contribute to losing weight, they also have inflammatory properties that prevent the resistance of insulin.

Seeds like chia seeds, pumpkin seeds, flaxseed, etc. are rich in fiber and omega-3fatty acids, and they lower the triglycerides and increase the good HDL cholesterol level which will help you reverse diabetes.

Legumes like lentils, chickpeas and beans are the perfect carbohydrate source. Due to their resistant starch, abundant fiber and moderate protein the release of glucose into your bloodstream can be significantly reduced.

Fruit like kiwi, berries, melon and oranges that are low in sugar will minimize glycemic effects. Rich in antioxidants and fiber, fresh fruits also contribute to reversing diabetes.

Vinegar decreases the glucose levels in your blood. A study has shown that two tablespoons of vinegar taken before each meal lowers your blood sugar for 25 %.

Besides these power foods, make sure to include fish that is high in omega 3-fatty acids, coconut and red palm oil, grass-fed beef and raw cheese to your diet.

Another healthy diet tips that will help you reverse diabetes:

- Make sure to include at least 1 ounce of fiber per day from high fiber foods that will slow down the glucose absorption.

- Sprinkle your cooked food with herbs like parsley and turmeric that will balance your blood sugar.

- Make a rainbow-colored selection of fruit and vegetables for each daily intake.

- Never skip breakfast. Missing the most important meal of the day will raise the glucose levels in your blood for the rest of the day.

- When you crave sugar, reach for some protein-packed food instead. A hard-boiled egg perhaps is a perfect way to charge your batteries.

- Be creative. Make new and tropical salads with leafy greens, berries, and citrus fruit and enjoy that zesty deliciousness while keeping your cells sensitive to insulin.

BOOKS BY LEE DOUGLAS

www.ingramcontent.com/pod-product-compliance
Lightning Source LLC
Chambersburg PA
CBHW060643290526
45793CB00001B/370